Exfoliate, Refresh and Replenish Your Skin

Over 20 of the Best Homemade Body Scrub Recipes for Your Skin

BY

Jenny Kings

Copyright 2019 Jenny Kings

License Notes

No part of this Book can be reproduced in any form or by any means including print, electronic, scanning or photocopying unless prior permission is granted by the author.

All ideas, suggestions and guidelines mentioned here are written for informative purposes. While the author has taken every possible to ensure accuracy, all readers are advised to follow information at their own risk. The author cannot be held responsible for personal and/or commercial damages in case of misinterpreting and misunderstanding any part of this Book

Table of Contents

Homemade Body Scrub Recipes 6

Body Scrub Recipes for Beginners 7

(1) Simple Sugar Scrub 8

(2) Lavender and Vanilla Brown Sugar Scrub 10

(3) Sugared Banana Body Scrub 12

(4) Simple Salt Body Scrub 14

(5) Tasty Chocolate Brown Sugar Scrub 16

Seasonal Body Scrub Recipes 18

(6) Gingerbread Body Scrub 19

(7) Facial Scrub for the Winter 21

(8) Spicy Pumpkin Sugar Scrub 24

(9) Summer's Over Sugared Tomato Scrub 26

(10) Hot Chocolate Body Scrub 28

Self-Care Body Scrub Recipes......................30

(11) Sensitive Skin Body Scrub...................31

(12) Pain Relieving Body Scrub 33

(13) Anti-Aging Body Scrub 36

(14) Clear Skin Body Scrub 38

(15) Daily Face Scrub............................40

Body Scrub Recipes for the Whole Family 43

(16) Almond Orange Body Scrub...................44

(17) Java Mint Body Scrub 46

(18) Mint Green Tea Body Scrub.................48

(19) Coffee Body Scrub 51

(20) Sugared Peach Body Scrub 53

Miscellaneous Body Scrub Recipes 55

(21) Lavender Foot Scrub 56

(22) The Stinker Foot Scrub.................................... 58

(23) Nourishing Lip Scrub..................................... 61

(24) Lemon Foot Scrub 63

(25) Two-Ingredient Coffee Lip Scrub 66

Author's Afterthoughts 68

Homemade Body Scrub Recipes

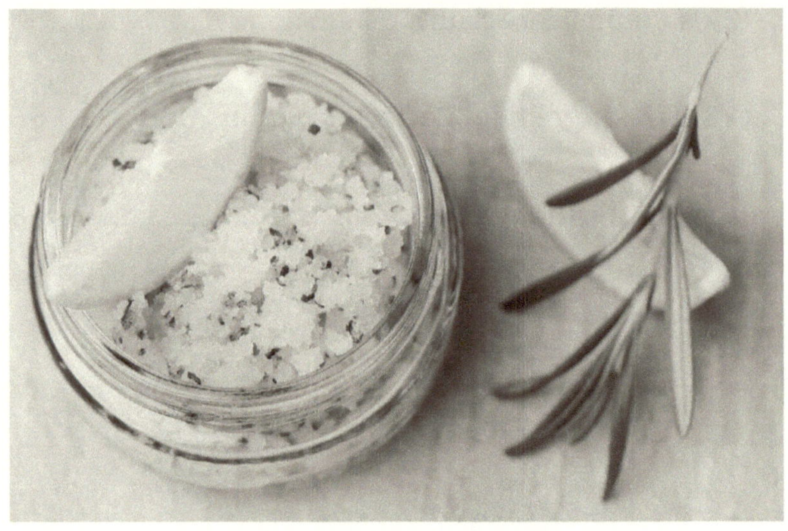

ooooooooooooooooooooooooooooooooooooooo

Body Scrub Recipes for Beginners

oooooooooooooooooooooooooooooooooooooooo

(1) Simple Sugar Scrub

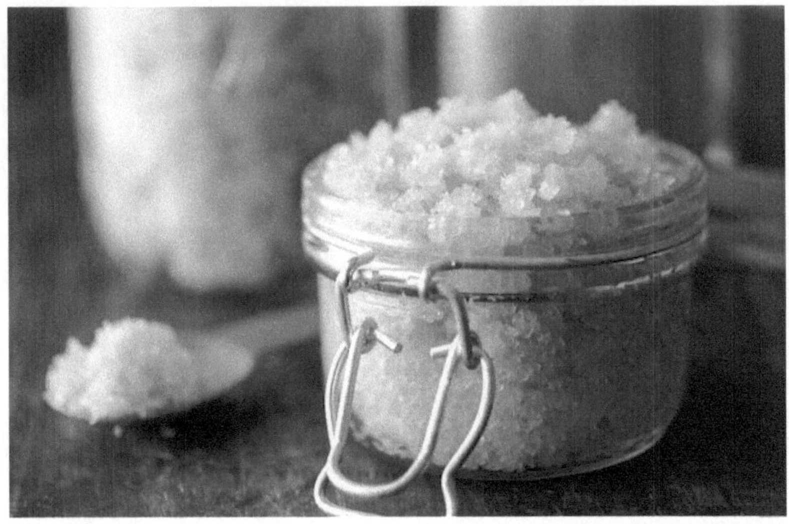

This recipe is the most basic of the sugar scrubs, which makes it a great starting point for beginners.

Makes: ¼ cup

Preparation Time: 3 to 5 minutes

List of Ingredients:

- ¼ cup granulated sugar
- ¼ cup olive oil, extra-virgin
- 2 drops essential oil, optional

OOOOOOOOOOOOOOOOOOOOOOOOOOOOOOOOOOOO

Procedure:

1: Place the sugar in a small bowl and drizzle the olive oil over top.

2: Using a spoon, combine the two ingredients together. Mix in the essential oil, if using, until all ingredients are well combined.

3: Store the sugar scrub in an airtight container for up to a month.

(2) Lavender and Vanilla Brown Sugar Scrub

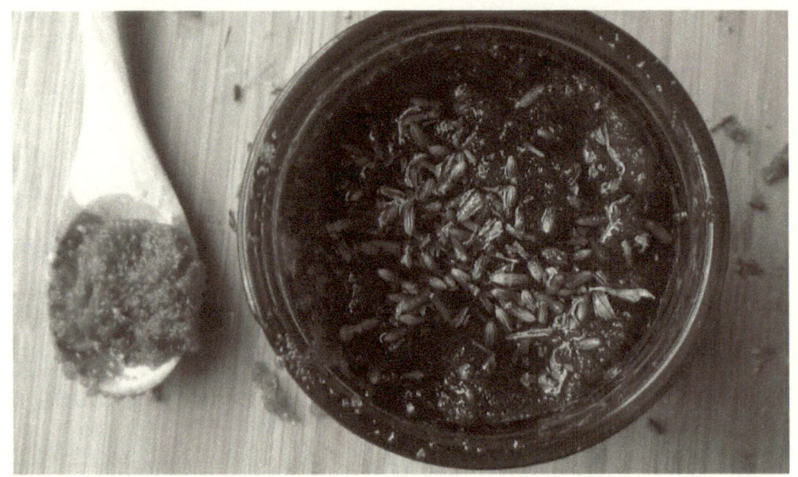

This body scrub recipes uses brown sugar as its base, with the addition of lavender essential oil and vanilla extract.

Makes: ¼ cup

Preparation Time: 3 to 5 minutes

List of Ingredients:

- ¼ cup brown sugar, packed
- ¼ cup olive oil, extra-virgin
- 3 drops vanilla extract, pure
- 2 drops lavender essential oil

OOOOOOOOOOOOOOOOOOOOOOOOOOOOOOOOOOOOOOO

Procedure:

1: Place the packed brown sugar into a bowl. Break up any clumps with a wooden spoon.

2: Drizzle the olive oil over top the brown sugar. Mix until well combined.

3: Mix in the pure vanilla extract, as well as the lavender essential oil until thoroughly combined.

4: Transfer the brown sugar body scrub to an airtight container. It should keep for up to a month.

(3) Sugared Banana Body Scrub

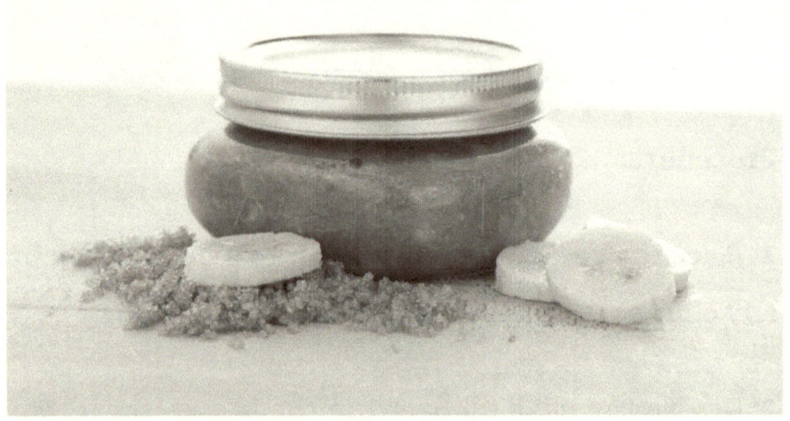

This sugared banana body scrub recipe works best when you use bananas that are overly ripe and are starting to turn brown. This is when the banana flavor is strong.

Makes: about ¼ to 1/3 cup

Preparation Time: 3 to 4 minutes

List of Ingredients:

- 3 tbsp. sugar, granulated
- 1 banana, extra ripe
- ¼ tsp. vanilla extract, pure

OOOOOOOOOOOOOOOOOOOOOOOOOOOOOOOOOOOOOOOO

Procedure:

1: Place the sugar in a bowl. Set the peeled banana on top of the granulated sugar.

2: Mash the banana into the sugar until well combined. Add in the vanilla extract and mash once again until all the ingredients are mixed into one another.

3: Spoon the body scrub into an airtight container. It should keep for up to a month.

(4) Simple Salt Body Scrub

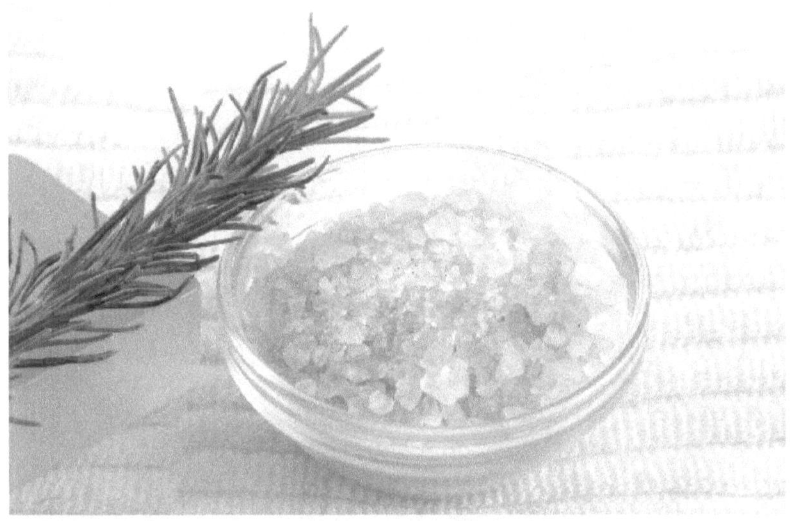

This basic body scrub is similar to the one above except it uses salt instead of sugar.

Makes: ½ cup

Preparation Time: 4 to 6 minutes

List of Ingredients:

- ½ cup sea salt
- ¼ cup olive oil, extra-virgin
- 2 drops essential oil, optional

OOOOOOOOOOOOOOOOOOOOOOOOOOOOOOOOOOOO

Procedure:

1: Mix the sea salt and oil together until well combined. Add in the essential oil if using.

2: Once the mixture is thoroughly mixed, transfer to an airtight container. The salt scrub should keep for up to a month.

(5) Tasty Chocolate Brown Sugar Scrub

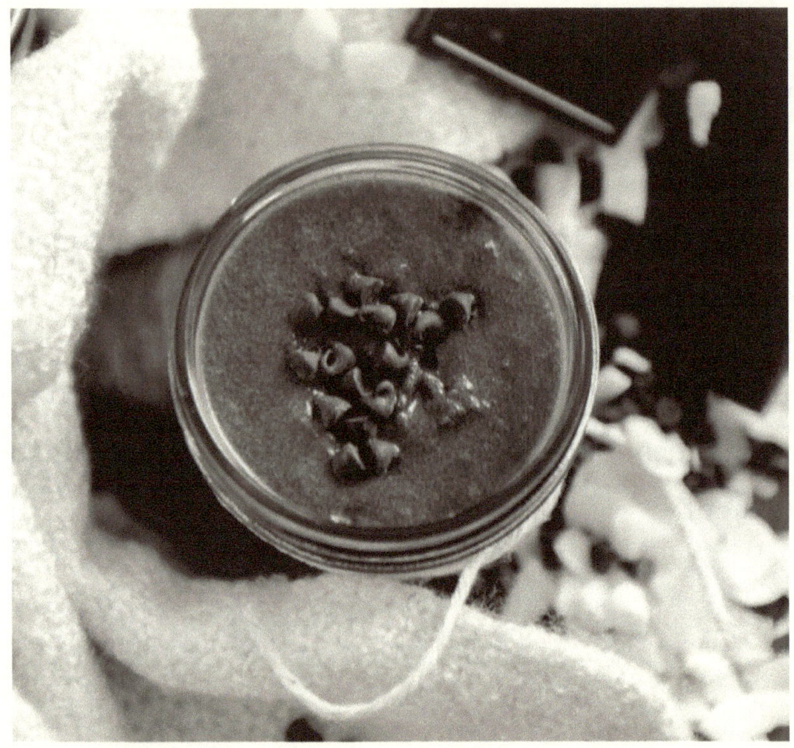

The addition of cocoa powder gives this brown sugar body scrub recipe a tasty chocolate flavor.

Makes: about ¾ cup

Preparation Time: 4 minutes

List of Ingredients:

- ½ cup brown sugar, packed
- ¼ cup cocoa powder, unsweetened
- 1 cup coconut oil, melted

OOOOOOOOOOOOOOOOOOOOOOOOOOOOOOOOOOOOOOO

Procedure:

1: Whisk together the packed brown sugar and the unsweetened cocoa powder, making sure you break up any clumps. Once the mixture is well combined continue onto the next step.

2: Drizzle the melted coconut oil overtop the mixture and stir until the oil is evenly distributed and mixed in.

3: Spoon the chocolate sugar body scrub into an airtight container. Keep in a cool, dry location for up to a month.

Seasonal Body Scrub Recipes

ooooooooooooooooooooooooooooooooooooooo

(6) Gingerbread Body Scrub

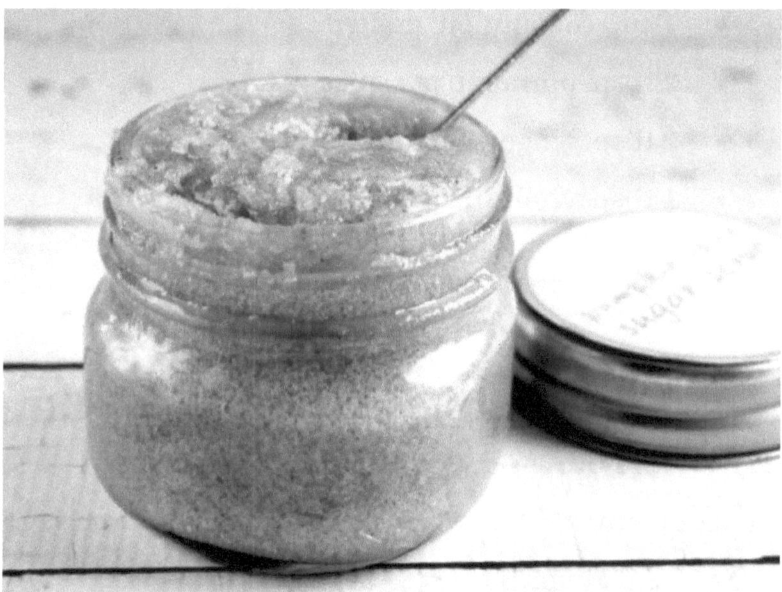

Who doesn't love some gingerbread cookies during the Holidays? This body scrub features brown sugar and has an aroma that will make you think someone is baking gingerbread cookies.

Makes: about 2 cups

Preparation Time: 3 to 4 minutes

List of Ingredients:

- 2 cups brown sugar, packed
- 1 cup coconut oil, melted
- 2 tbsp. pumpkin pie spice
- 2 tbsp. ginger, ground
- 1 tbsp. vitamin E oil

OOOOOOOOOOOOOOOOOOOOOOOOOOOOOOOOOOOOOOOO

Procedure:

1: Pour the brown sugar into a bowl. Use a whisk to break up any lumps. Mix in the pumpkin pie spice and the ground ginger.

2: Stir the melted coconut oil and the vitamin E oil into the mixture until thoroughly combined.

3: Transfer the mixture into an airtight container and store in a cool, dark location for 3 to 6 weeks.

(7) Facial Scrub for the Winter

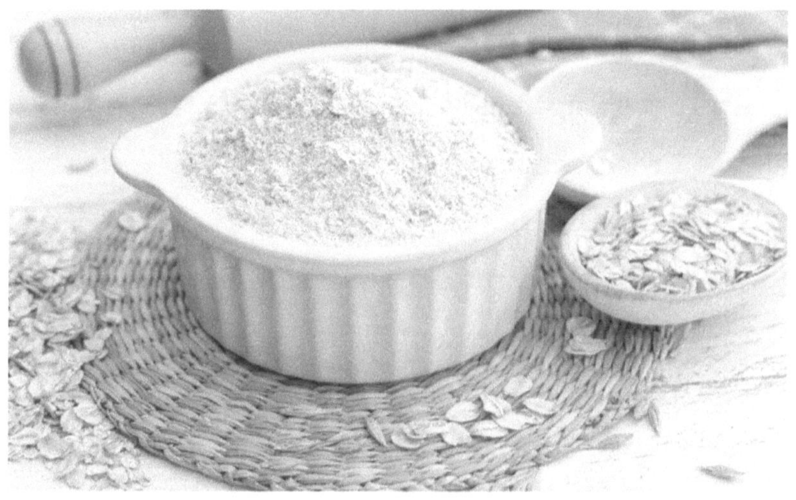

This facial scrub will help keep your skin looking its best, even during those harsh winter months.

Makes: about ¼ to ½ cup

Preparation Time: 6 minutes

List of Ingredients:

- ¼ cup finely ground oats
- 1/8 cup shredded coconut, unsweetened
- 1/3 cup white rice flour
- 1 tbsp. kaolin clay
- 1 tbsp. neem powder
- 2 tbsp. chamomile
- 2 tbsp. calendula
- 10 drops chamomile essential oil
- 10 drops rose essential oil
- 15 drops rose hip seed essential oil

OOOOOOOOOOOOOOOOOOOOOOOOOOOOOOOOOOOOOO

Procedure:

1: Place the shredded coconut, oats, chamomile and calendula into a food processor. Pulse the ingredients until they are finely ground.

2: Transfer the finely ground mixture into a bowl.

3: Stir the kaolin clay, neem powder, and white rice flour into the finely ground mixture from 2.

4: Mix the rose essential oil, chamomile essential oil, and rose hip seed oil into the dry mixture from 3.

5: Transfer the facial scrub to an airtight container and store in a cool, dry area for up to 4 months.

6: To use, place about a tsp. of the facial scrub into your palm and add a couple of drops of water. Spread the scrub over your face and, in a circular motion, gently scrub the mixture into your skin. Rinse your face with water and dry with a clean towel.

(8) Spicy Pumpkin Sugar Scrub

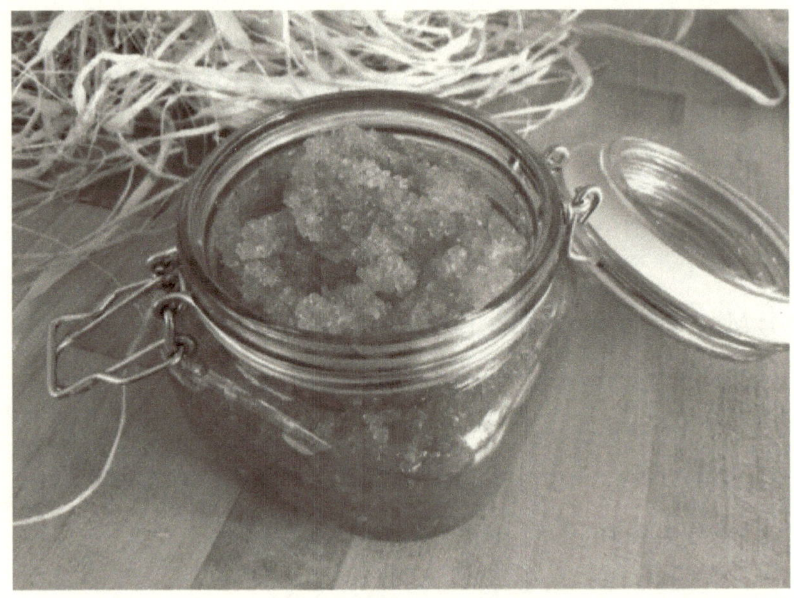

A staple for the autumn season, pumpkin works well in just about anything, including this spicy sugar scrub recipe.

Makes: about 2 cups

Preparation Time: 3 minutes

List of Ingredients:

- 2 cups brown sugar, packed
- ½ cup granulated sugar
- ½ tsp. nutmeg
- 1 tsp. pumpkin pie spice
- 1 tsp. cinnamon
- ½ cup sweet almond oil

OOOOOOOOOOOOOOOOOOOOOOOOOOOOOOOOOOOO

Procedure:

1: Stir together the packed brown sugar and the granulated sugar until well mixed. Make sure you break up any lumps in the sugar mixture.

2: Whisk the nutmeg, pumpkin pie spice and cinnamon into the sugar mixture.

3: Drizzle the sweet almond oil over top the mixture and mash with a spoon until the oil is completely disturbed throughout the mixture.

4: Transfer the body scrub to an airtight container. Store the container in the fridge for about 6 weeks.

(9) Summer's Over Sugared Tomato Scrub

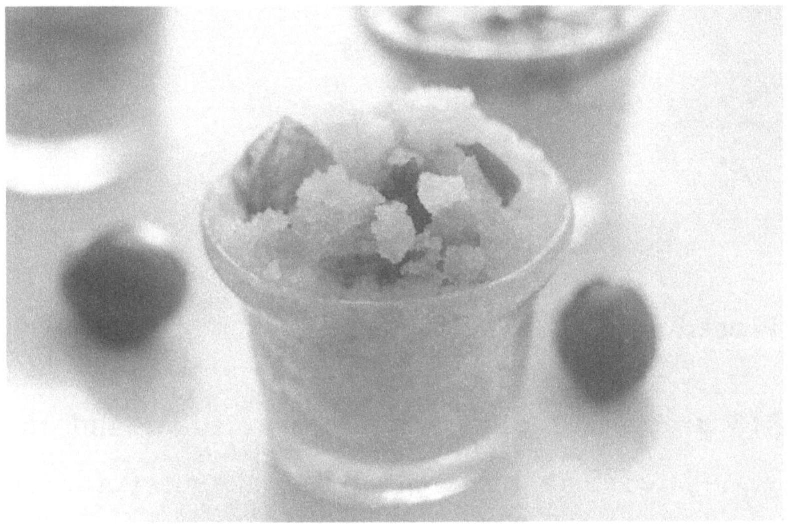

This tomato sugar body scrub is a great way to end the summer season and prepare your skin for the winter months.

Makes: about 2 cups

Preparation Time: 5 minutes

List of Ingredients:

- 2 cups sugar, granulated
- 1 tomato, diced
- ¾ cup olive oil
- 15 drops essential oil, citronella or lemon

OOOOOOOOOOOOOOOOOOOOOOOOOOOOOOOOOOOOOOOO

Procedure:

1: Place the diced tomato into a bowl and roughly chop it into tiny, fine pieces. The tomato should have a consistency close to mush.

2: Pour the sugar on top of the mushed tomato and mix the two ingredients together. Add the olive oil, followed by the essential oil, and combined.

3: Transfer the mixture into an airtight container. Place the container in the fridge and store for up to 3 weeks.

(10) Hot Chocolate Body Scrub

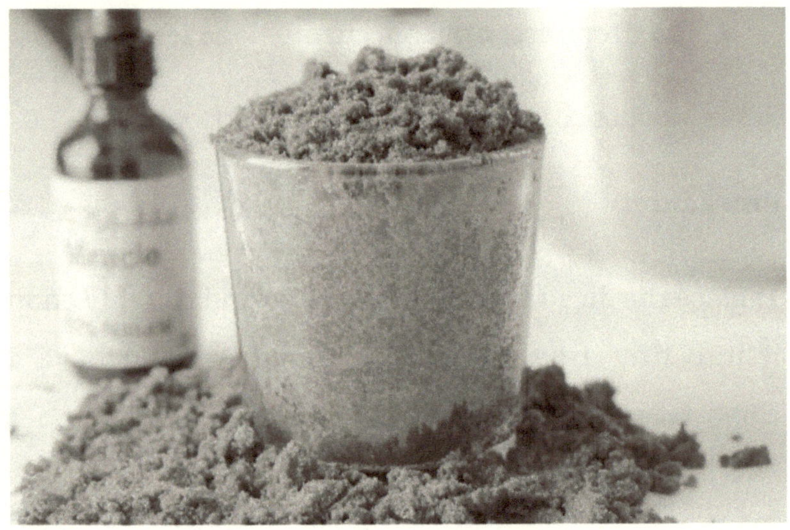

This sugar body scrub is the perfect way to "warm up" during those winter months and will leave your skin smelling like a nice cup of hot cocoa.

Makes: about 1 cup

Preparation Time: 4 minutes

List of Ingredients:

- 3 tbsp. cocoa powder, unsweetened
- 1 cup brown sugar, packed
- 1 tsp. vanilla
- ½ cup sweet almond oil

OOOOOOOOOOOOOOOOOOOOOOOOOOOOOOOOOOOOOOO

Procedure:

1: Combine the cocoa powder with the brown sugar. Add in the vanilla and stir for a few seconds.

2: Drizzle the sweet almond oil over top of the mixture and stir until well combined.

3: Transfer the body scrub to an airtight container and store in a cool, dry location for about 4 weeks.

Self-Care Body Scrub Recipes

(11) Sensitive Skin Body Scrub

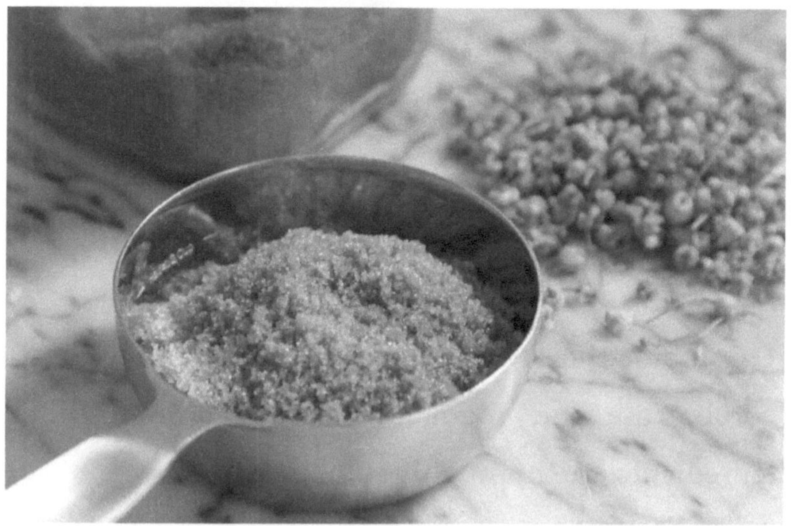

This body scrub is perfect for those who suffering with sensitive skin. It utilizes chamomile, rose and neroli essential oil to gently cleanse and soothe skin.

Makes: about 1 cup

Preparation Time: 3 to 4 minutes

List of Ingredients:

- 1 cup sugar, granulated
- ½ cup oil, olive or sunflower
- 2 drops neroli essential oil
- 4 drops rose essential oil
- 6 drops chamomile essential oil

ooooooooooooooooooooooooooooooooooooo

Procedure:

1: Combine the sugar and the oil together. Add in the neroli, rose and chamomile essential oil until all ingredients are thoroughly combined.

2: Transfer the sugar scrub to an airtight container. The scrub should keep for up to a month.

(12) Pain Relieving Body Scrub

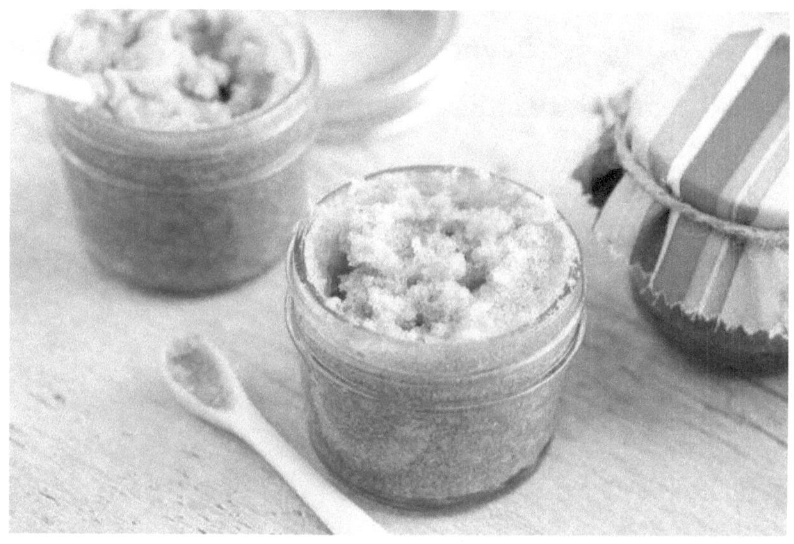

This salt body scrub helps to relive pain associated with muscles and joints.

Makes: about 1 cup

Preparation Time: 5 to 6 minutes

List of Ingredients:

- 1 cup sea salt
- ½ tsp. ground cinnamon
- ½ cup coconut oil, melted
- 5 drops eucalyptus essential oil
- 5 drops lavender essential oil

ooooooooooooooooooooooooooooooooooooooo

Procedure:

1: Mix the sea salt with the ground cinnamon. Once the two are thoroughly combined, drizzle the melted coconut oil overtop and mash together with a spoon.

2: Add in the eucalyptus essential oil and the lavender essential oil and mash with the spoon until the essential oils are well combined with the other ingredients.

3: Transfer the salt scrub to an airtight container. It should keep for up to a month.

4: To use, gently rub the scrub over the painful sore joints or muscles. Wait for several minutes and then rinse the scrub off with water and pat dry with a clean towel.

(13) Anti-Aging Body Scrub

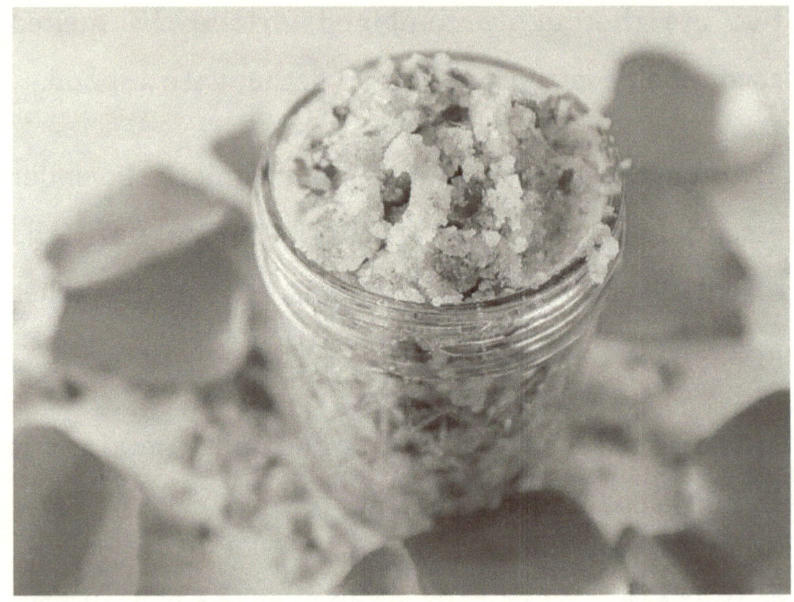

This body scrub recipe features rosehip oil, which has a naturally high amount of vitamin A. Studies have shown that vitamin A can help to increase collagen and elastin, as well as acting as an anti-aging for the skin.

Makes: about 1 cup

Preparation Time: 5 minutes

List of Ingredients:

- 1 cup sugar, granulated
- ½ cup oil, olive or coconut
- 6 drops rosehip essential oil
- 1 tbsp. rose flowers, dried (optional)

OOOOOOOOOOOOOOOOOOOOOOOOOOOOOOOOOOOOOOOO

Procedure:

1: In a small mixing bowl, mix the sugar, rosehip essential oil and oil together until well combined. If using dried rose flowers, mix them into the concoction as well.

2: Transfer the anti-aging body scrub into an airtight container and keep for up to a month.

3: When ready to use, rub the body scrub gently into wrinkles, dry skin areas, and age spots.

(14) Clear Skin Body Scrub

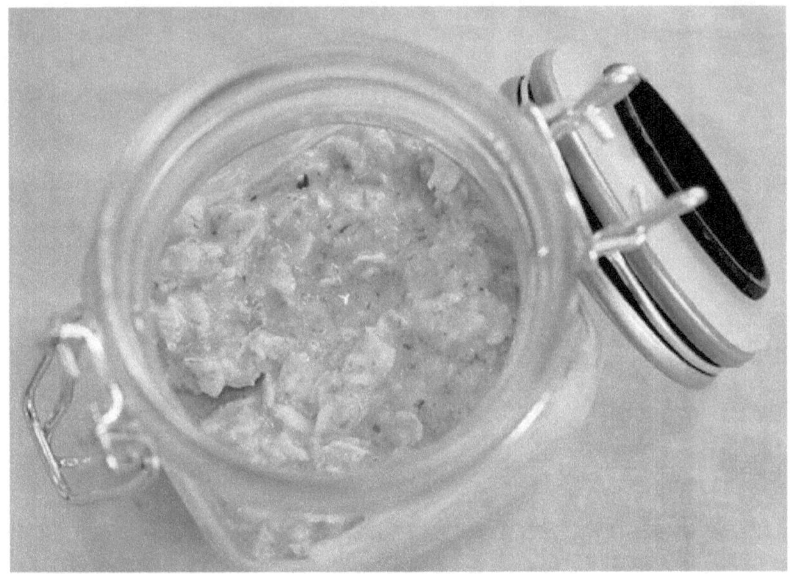

This body scrub helps to naturally keep your skin clear while keeping acne at bay. What's even better is that it can be used on any part of your body where you are battling a flare-up of acne.

Makes: about 1 cup

Preparation Time: 4 to 5 minutes

List of Ingredients:

- 1 cup oats, finely ground
- ½ cup distilled water
- 5 drops lavender essential oil
- 10 drops lemon essential oil
- 10 drops cypress essential oil

OOOOOOOOOOOOOOOOOOOOOOOOOOOOOOOOOOOOOOO

Procedure:

1: In a small bowl, mix the oats with the distilled water. Stir in the lavender, lemon, and cypress essential oil until well combined.

2: Transfer the body scrub to an airtight container. When ready to use, massage a bit of the scrub into the problem area before rinsing it off with water and then patting yourself dry with a clean towel.

(15) Daily Face Scrub

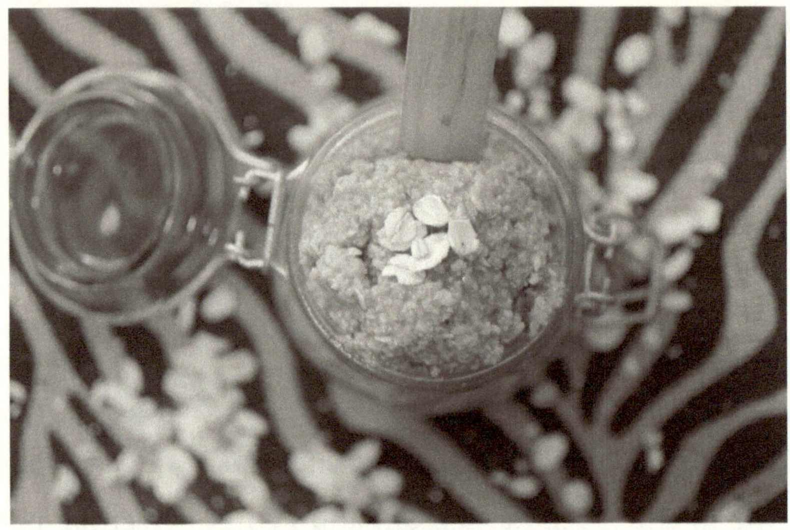

The ingredients in this face scrub recipe will vary depending on the type of skin you have. You simply mix the base ingredients together and then add the remaining ingredients for your specific skin type.

Makes: 4 to 6 tsp.

Preparation Time: 4 minutes

List of Ingredients:

Base Ingredients:

- 1 tsp. ground almond meal
- 1 tsp. ground oats
- 1 tsp. powdered milk
- ½ tsp. distilled water

Combination Skin Ingredients:

- 2 tbsp. cornmeal
- 2 tbsp. dried and finely ground chamomile
- 5 drops lavender essential oil

Dry Skin Ingredients:

- 2 tbsp. powdered milk, full fat
- 2 tbsp. finely ground calendula
- 5 drops chamomile essential oil

Oily Skin Ingredients:

- 2 tbsp. sea salt, finely ground
- 2 tbsp. dried and ground peppermint
- 5 drops rosemary essential oil

Procedure:

1: Mix all the base ingredients together in a bowl.

2: Choose the type of skin you have and add in the corresponding ingredients to the base mixture from 1.

3: Combine until all the desired ingredients are well mixed. Store in an airtight container.

4: Use every morning to keep your skin fresh, clean and looking its best.

Body Scrub Recipes for the Whole Family

OOOOOOOOOOOOOOOOOOOOOOOOOOOOOOOOOOOOO

(16) Almond Orange Body Scrub

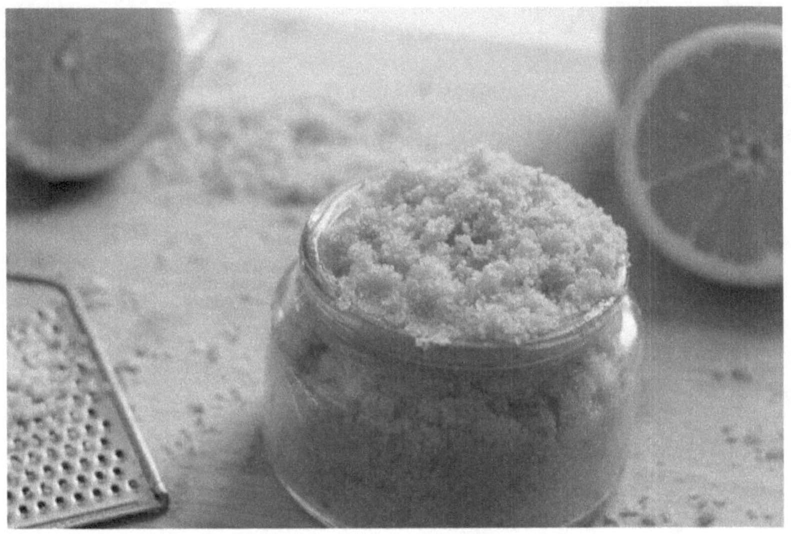

This body scrub recipe doesn't use sugar or salt as the exfoliator. Instead it utilizes almonds!

Makes: about 1 cup

Preparation Time: 5 minutes

List of Ingredients:

- 1 cup grapeseed oil
- 1 orange peel
- Handful of shelled almonds, unsalted

OOOOOOOOOOOOOOOOOOOOOOOOOOOOOOOOOOOOOOO

Procedure:

1: Place the grapeseed oil, orange peel and almonds into a food processor. Pulse the mixture until it has a gritty and thick constancy.

2: Scoop the mixture out of the food processor and into an airtight container. The body scrub will last up to 1 month if stored in a cool, dry location away from direct heat and direct sunlight.

(17) Java Mint Body Scrub

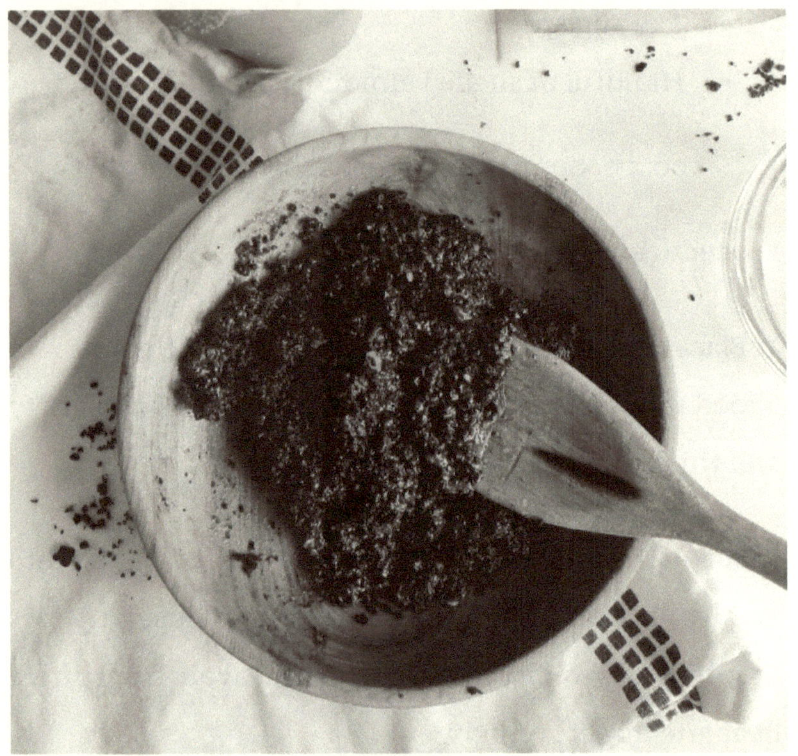

This masculine-scented body scrub can be used by anyone who doesn't want their skin left with a floral or fruity fragrance.

Makes: about 1 cup

Preparation Time: 13 to 15 minutes

List of Ingredients:

- ½ cup sugar, granulated
- ½ cup coffee grounds, unused
- ¼ cup distilled water, hot
- ¼ cup sweet almond oil
- 15 drops peppermint essential oil

ooooooooooooooooooooooooooooooooooooooooo

Procedure:

1: In a small bowl, combine the sugar and the coffee grounds together. Gradually stir in the hot, distilled water. Let the mixture sit for about 10 minutes before continuing.

2: Stir in the sweet almond oil, followed by the peppermint essential oil. Once the mixture is well combined, transfer it to an airtight container.

3: Store the body scrub in a cool, dry location for up to one month.

(18) Mint Green Tea Body Scrub

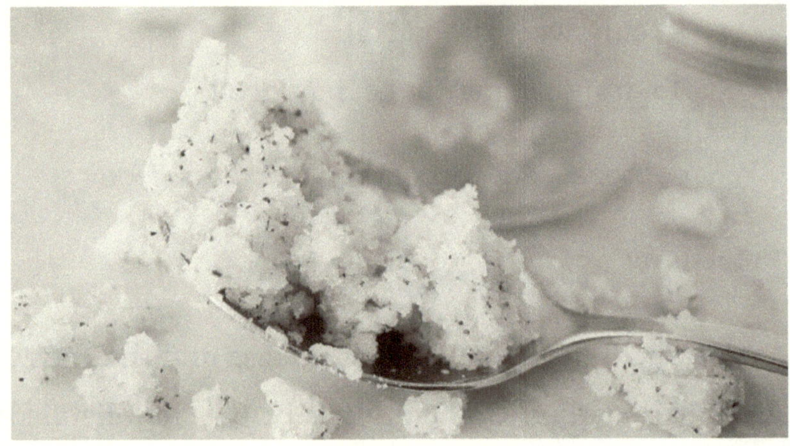

This minty green tea body scrub is the perfect way to start your day and will leave your skin feeling refreshed.

Makes: about 1 cup

Preparation Time: 5 to 6 minutes

List of Ingredients:

- 1 cup sugar, granulated
- 3 tbsp. Epsom salts
- 2 bags green tea
- 2 bags mint tea
- 2 tbsp. olive oil
- 2 tbsp. pure honey
- 4 drops vitamin E oil, optional

OOOOOOOOOOOOOOOOOOOOOOOOOOOOOOOOOOOOOOO

Procedure:

1: Mix the sugar and the Epsom salt together in a mixing bowl.

2: Tear open all four of the tea bags. Pour the tea into the mixing bowl from 1. Stir until the ingredients are well combined.

3: Stir in the olive oil, followed by the honey. Once the mixture is well combined, add the vitamin E oil, if using.

4: Transfer the mixture into an airtight container. It will last up to a month.

(19) Coffee Body Scrub

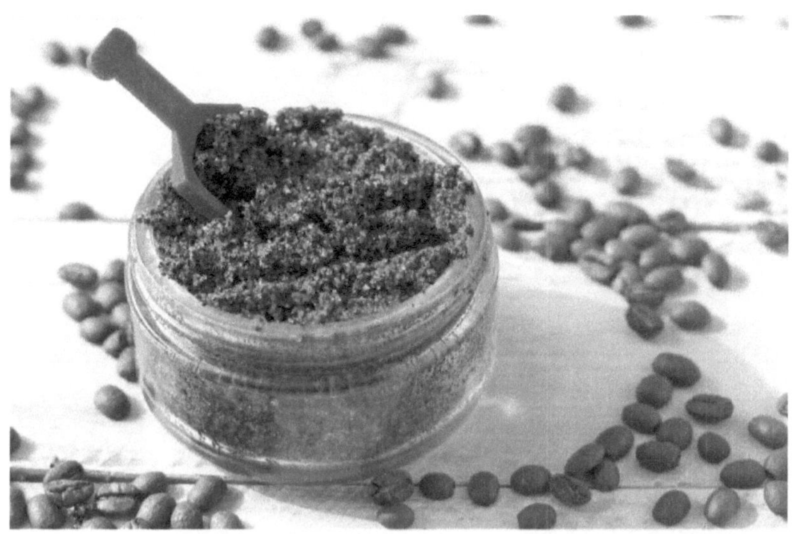

This brown sugar body scrub doesn't feature a feminine scent and you can choose the desired essential oil to fit the fragrance you prefer.

Makes: about ½ to ¾ cup

Preparation Time: 4 to 5 minutes

List of Ingredients:

- ¼ cup brown sugar, packed
- ¼ cup coffee grounds, unused
- ¼ cup sea salt
- ½ cup oil, coconut or olive
- 25 drops essential oi, such as sandalwood, oakmoss, spruce, balsam, or basil

OOOOOOOOOOOOOOOOOOOOOOOOOOOOOOOOOOOOOO

Procedure:

1: In a mixing bowl, stir together the sugar, coffee grounds and salt until well mixed. Add in the oil and mix until combined.

2: Stir in the desired essential oil. Once the mixture is thoroughly combined, transfer to body scrub into an airtight container. Store the container for up to a month in a cool, dry area.

3: To use, gently rub the body scrub onto your skin in a circular motion. Rinse the scrub off with water and pat dry with a clean towel.

(20) Sugared Peach Body Scrub

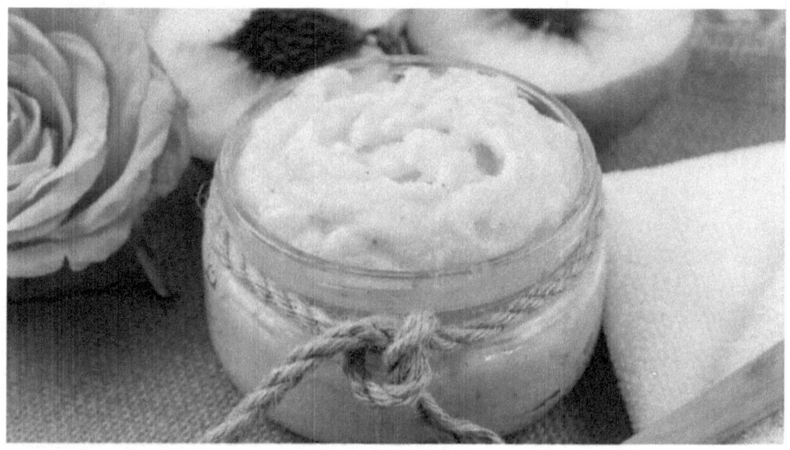

This sugared peach body scrub leaves your skin lightly scented with a peachy aroma.

Makes: about 1 cup

Preparation Time: 3 to 4 minutes

List of Ingredients:

- 1 cup sugar, granulated
- ½ cup olive oil
- 3 drops peach essential oil

OOOOOOOOOOOOOOOOOOOOOOOOOOOOOOOOOOOOOOOO

Procedure:

1: Mix the sugar and olive oil together until well combined. Add the peach essential oil and stir.

2: Spoon the mixture into a glass jar and secure closed with the lid. Keep in a cool, dry location for up to a month.

Miscellaneous Body Scrub Recipes

OOOOOOOOOOOOOOOOOOOOOOOOOOOOOOOOOOOOOO

(21) Lavender Foot Scrub

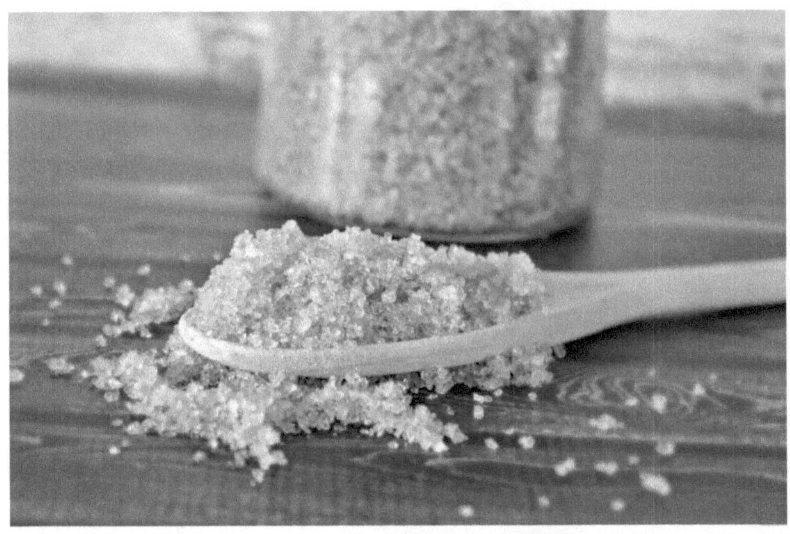

This foot scrub will leave your feet feeling soft and smooth with a pleasant lavender aroma.

Makes: about 1 cup

Preparation Time: 3 minutes

List of Ingredients:

- 1 cup salt, sea or Epsom
- 2 tbsp. dried lavender buds
- ½ cup olive oil
- 6 drops lavender essential oil

OOOOOOOOOOOOOOOOOOOOOOOOOOOOOOOOOOOOOO

Procedure:

1: Combine the salt with the dried lavender buds. Add in the olive oil, followed by the lavender essential oil. Stir until all the ingredients are well combined.

2: Spoon the foot scrub mixture into an airtight container and store in a cool, dry location.

3: To use, gently scrub the mixture into damp feet. Wait for several seconds before rinsing the scrub off and drying with a clean towel.

(22) The Stinker Foot Scrub

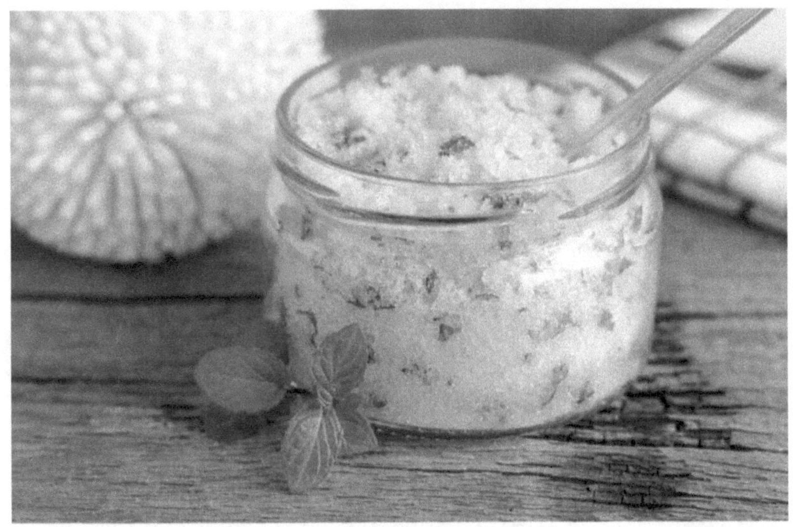

This foot scrub will help de-stink those feet! The tea tree essential oil helps to kill bacteria that is known to cause stinky feet.

Makes: about ½ cup

Preparation Time: 3 to 4 minutes

List of Ingredients:

- 2/3 cup Epsom salts
- 1/3 cup sugar, raw
- ½ tbsp. dried peppermint leaves
- 1 ½ tbsp. coconut oil, melted
- 5 drops peppermint essential oil
- 4 drops tea tree essential oil

OOOOOOOOOOOOOOOOOOOOOOOOOOOOOOOOOOOOOO

Procedure:

1: Mix the salt and sugar together. Add in the dried peppermint leaves and mix until evenly distributed.

2: Stir in the melted coconut oil, followed by the peppermint essential oil and the tea tree essential oil. Once all the ingredients are well combined, continue on with the remaining steps.

3: Transfer the foot scrub into an airtight container. Store in a cool, dry location for up to 1 month.

4: To use, gently scrub the mixture into damp feet. Wait for several seconds before rinsing the scrub off and drying with a clean towel.

(23) Nourishing Lip Scrub

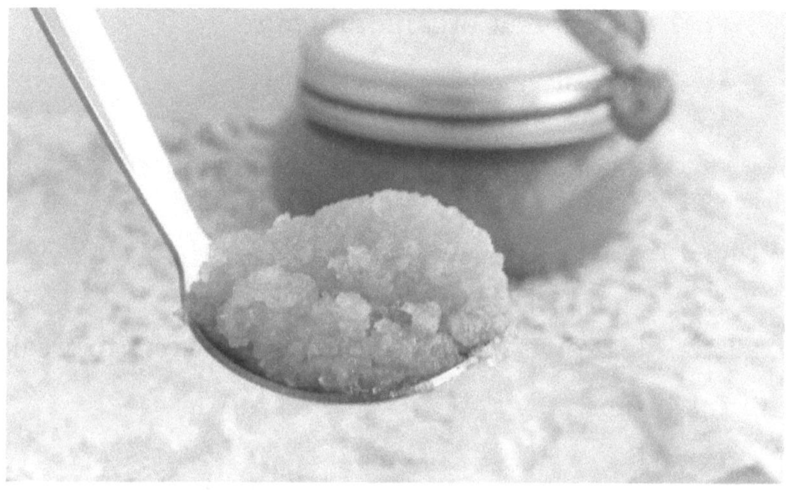

This lip scrub will not only leave your skin feeling soft, but it will also naturally moisturize them.

Makes: about 2 tbsp.

Preparation Time: 3 minutes

List of Ingredients:

- 1 tbsp. brown sugar, packed
- 1 tbsp. honey, organic and pure
- 1 tbsp. olive oil

OOOOOOOOOOOOOOOOOOOOOOOOOOOOOOOOOOOOOOOO

Procedure:

1: Place the brown sugar into a bowl. Use a fork to break up any lumps.

2: Using the fork, mix the honey and olive oil into the brown sugar.

3: Transfer the lip scrub to a small glass container. To use, rub a small amount of the scrub gently over your lips. Wait several seconds before rinsing the scrub off with water.

(24) Lemon Foot Scrub

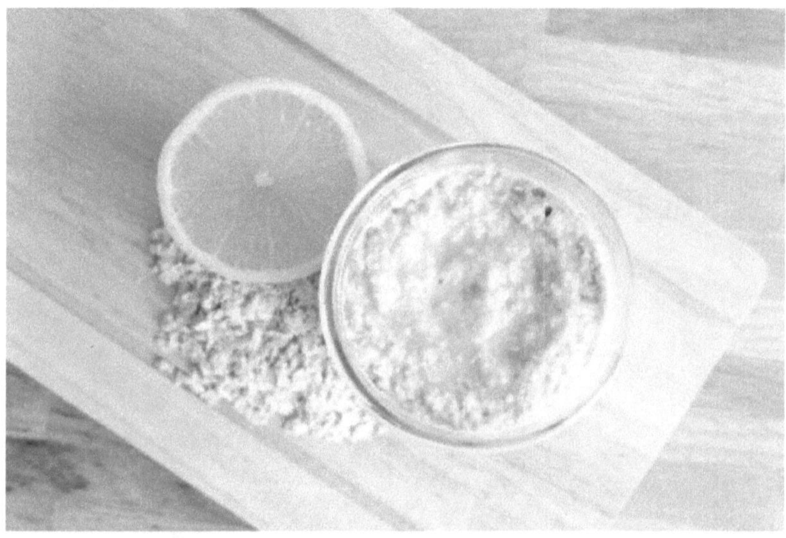

This lemon foot scrub leaves your feet feeling soft and revegetated.

Makes: about 1 cup

Preparation Time: 3 to 4 minutes

List of Ingredients:

- ½ cup cornmeal
- ½ cup oats
- 2 tbsp. sea salt
- 5 drops lemon essential oil
- Water

OOOOOOOOOOOOOOOOOOOOOOOOOOOOOOOOOOOOOOO

Procedure:

1: Process the oats in a food processor until they have a powder-like constancy. Transfer the oats to a mixing bowl.

2: Add the salt and cornmeal to the oats and stir until well combined. Mix in the lemon essential oil before continuing.

3: Add the water, a little at time, making sure to stir after each addition. You want to add just enough water so that the mixture has a paste-like consistency that is gritty.

4: Transfer the scrub to an airtight container and store for several weeks.

5: To use, gently scrub the mixture into damp feet. Wait for several seconds before rinsing the scrub off and drying with a clean towel.

(25) Two-Ingredient Coffee Lip Scrub

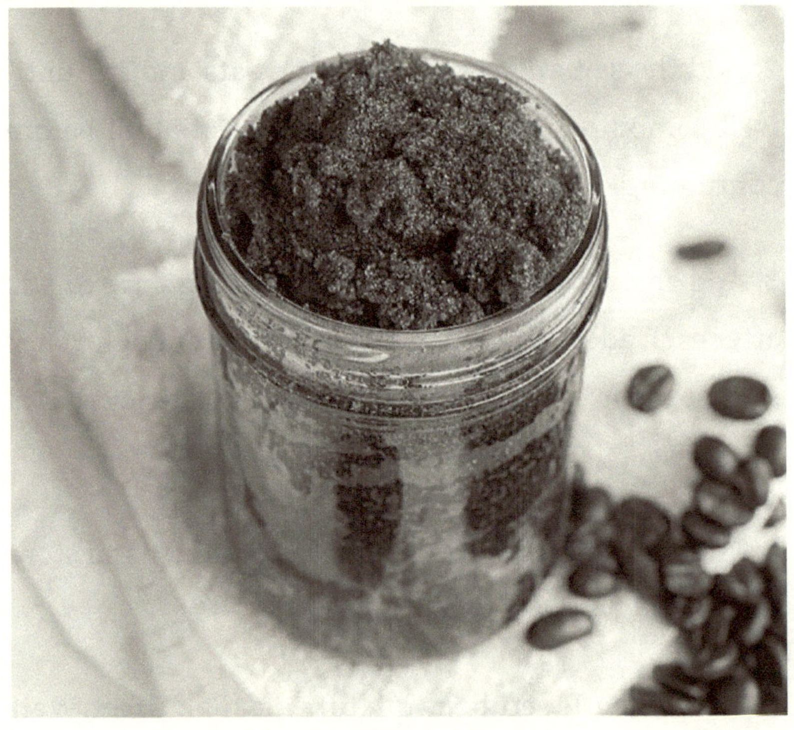

This maybe one of the easiest lip scrub recipes out there to make and it only requires two ingredients that you may just currently have in your pantry.

Makes: about 1 tbsp.

Preparation Time: 2 minutes

List of Ingredients:

- 1 tbsp. coffee grounds, unused
- 1 tbsp. olive oil

ooooooooooooooooooooooooooooooooooooo

Procedure:

1: Combine the coffee grounds with the olive oil until the ingredients are well mixed into one another.

2: Store the coffee lip scrub in a glass jar kept in a dry, cool location.

3: To use, gently scrub a small amount of the mixture onto your lips before wiping them clean with a damp cloth.

Author's Afterthoughts

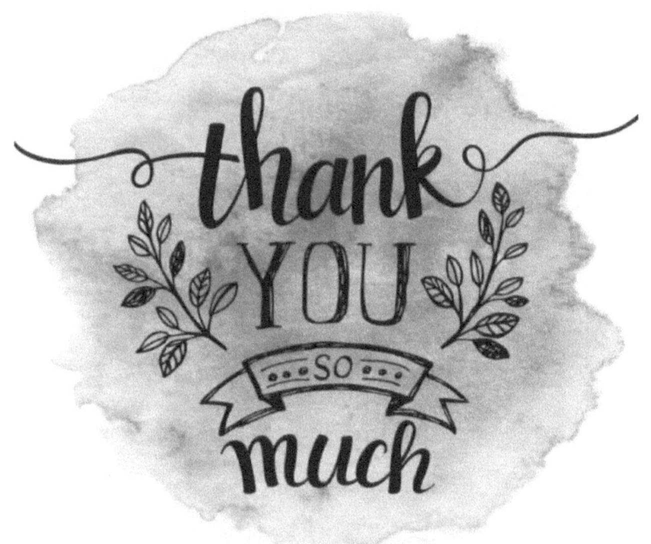

Thank you for reading my book. Your feedback is important to me. It would be greatly appreciated if you could please take a moment to REVIEW this book on Amazon so that we could make our next version better

Thanks!

Jenny Kings